Booze, Blow, and Pancakes

Breaking Free From the Shackles of Addiction

Yvette Salva

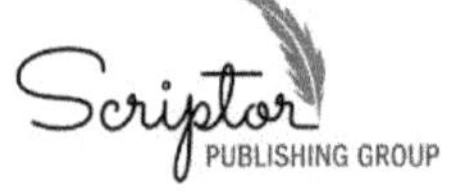
Scriptor
PUBLISHING GROUP

I dedicate this book to Dave, Mary Rose, and Steven.

To my best friend, Dave Salva
I am so honored to be a Salva, truly! You, and only you,
believed in me when no one else did. You took a chance on
me. I had nothing to offer you when we met except a few
good laughs and a big heart. You showed me how to live.
You showed me about family, you showed me about work
ethic, and you showed me what unconditional love is.
I am forever grateful.

To my beautiful daughter, Mary Rose, My "ride or die"
You saved my life in so many ways.
Thank you for always believing in me…
And I'm sorry you had to see your mommy
struggle with the food.
You give my life meaning and purpose…
The best job I ever did was to become a mom.
I'm so proud of the woman that you are becoming.
You are strong, courageous kind and
have a most beautiful heart.
You can be and do anything in this world.

To my beautiful son, Steven
My life is better because you are in it. You have the most
beautiful, kindest heart. I'm so grateful to be your mom.
Thank you for being my son. I love you so much.
You can do and be anything in this world.

Table of Contents

Introduction

When I first met Yvette, it was through a computer screen with 40 other faces. We were both upcoming life coaches in a six month online coaching program. All 40 of us basically got to know each other on a weekly basis from the neck up on Zoom. Later on, I actually found out that Yvette was already a life coach and that she took the course mainly to improve her skills.

It wasn't long into the program where everyone got to know more about Yvette and her past addictions. She told her shortened story numerous times, as it's important to her, and she tells it to help others.

About halfway through the program, Yvette and I did some practice coaching sessions together as well as got to know each other much more, still online as we live almost 1000 miles apart. After a while, I got to know Yvette and hear her story on a much deeper level. And what an amazing story it is. She has gone through so much and has hit the very low of lows to come out of it as such a beautiful woman inside and out. She is now a thriving woman, mother, coach, and friend to so many. After finally meeting Yvette in person, sitting with her talking face-to- face, it's easy to see that she is so genuine and cares about helping others so much. I'm so glad that Yvette came into my life as she is just one of those people that lifts you up.

Yvette just loves to help people. She has a very large servant heart. One of the largest I have ever seen. From her personal training business to her life coaching business, to helping others grow their businesses and personal life, and just being a great friend to so many, and being an amazing mother to her two children, Yvette is just the kind of person you want to be around. She knows what she's good at and knows what she's not.

One of the reasons I agreed to help Yvette write this book is because she is so honest about her past. Yvette recovers out loud and wants you to do the same. She definitely does NOT want to be anonymous, as many that have gone through similar addictions try to hide that part of their life. Yvette has taken the shame out of addiction by speaking of her past experiences, through this book, her keynotes, and so many other coaching avenues.

Yvette talks about how she went from a homeless stripper living in her car, addicted to drugs and alcohol, to becoming an entrepreneur who's changing lives through fitness and mindset. Her mindset is all about growth and how she can improve herself to help others grow themselves. She is such an inspiration to me and to so many others. After helping her with this book, I know she can also help so many more.

Yvette is such an inspiration as she's always keeping her head down, moving forward, never taking her foot off the pedal. Take her story from this book and the lessons she gives you to heart as this book might just be the spark of light you need to save your own life.

~ Chad Cannon

Chapter 1

Secrets Keep You Sick

You might be wondering why I chose the title, *Booze, Blow, and Pancakes*, for this book. We all understand "booze" and most of us know what "blow" is, but you might be curious to find out what the pancakes have to do with it.

So, let me tell you.

Believe it or not, there was a time in my life when I had a love affair with pancakes. It wasn't because they tasted great. It's because I learned very quickly that they were one of the easiest foods to puke up. When they were covered with butter and syrup, they would come up so easily that I didn't have to spend hours gagging myself. Once I learned this secret, it didn't take long for pancakes to become my obsession, and they kept me in the grips of addiction with bulimia for more than 30 years.

But let's start back at the beginning so you can see how my journey unfolded.

My family moved to America from Spain when I was in seventh grade. It was a complete culture shock at a very vulnerable time in my life, and I definitely didn't fit in. My mom is black, and my dad is white. Back then, there was a lot of prejudice against mixed races. It's so different now with celebrities like Beyonce, J-Lo and Drake who have made it cool to be brown. But back then, the kids called me "spic" and "Oreo," and told me to go back to Spain.

I clearly didn't look like the American girls, and I didn't want to have my black hair. I didn't want to be a foreigner in this country. And I didn't want to be brown! Every day I came home from school crying, telling my parents that I wanted to go back to Spain, change my name to Cindy and get a "Farrah Fawcett" haircut. The obsession with my appearance began there, but even if I had changed my name and my haircut, none of that would have changed how I felt on the inside. The bottom line was that I felt like dog shit… all the time!

I soon recognized that weight loss was the social currency with all the girls in school. So, that became my goal, and that is where the downward spiral began. I learned pretty quickly that whatever you put your mind to, you will achieve! I started running after school and began to lose weight. Since I thought I looked good, I kept running. And by the end of 8th grade, I was down to 79 pounds. At the same time, I also realized that becoming a cheerleader was a way to get boys, and so that became the second goal I achieved. Combined with losing weight, I now had social currency, but the fallout was that I had become addicted to weight loss. By the time I was a freshman in high school, I had entered my first treatment center.

The rehab center I went to was a locked unit, which is crazy, when you think about it. The rest of the facility was filled with drug addicts and alcoholics, and here I was, a freshman in high school with an eating disorder. I just wanted to be in the non-locked unit with the cool kids. Even though there were still drug addicts and alcoholics there, I still wished I could be there instead of where I was. Ironically, a few years later, I actually did end up in that unit. But at this point, I was still a freshman in high school. And at that moment it felt like once again, I didn't fit in, and once again, I was in a place I didn't want to be, wishing I was somewhere else.

Soon after I was released from the treatment center, I went to the mall with my girlfriend. We were going to buy some Dexatrim. Those of you who grew up in the '80s might remember the little yellow tablets that were supposed to help you lose weight. After we bought them, she said, "Let's go to the bathroom. I'm going to throw up my dinner."

Standing in the bathroom of the Livingston Mall, surrounded by all that white tile and bright, fluorescent lighting, I couldn't quite grasp what she was saying. As she backed into the first stall, I asked her, "How are you going to do that?"

Without responding, she turned around, stuck her fingers down her throat and threw up her spaghetti dinner. I will never forget it. I thought about it all the way home. I suddenly had a dirty little secret, and I couldn't wait to try it. The next day after school, I thought, I'm going to figure out how to do that, too. So I ate some Oreos—not just two cookies, but two entire sleeves of them! And I swallowed them down with so much milk! Then I went to the bathroom and tried to throw up. It didn't work. But I wasn't going to give up that easily. I decided to get creative and gagged myself with every utensil I could think of, even a freaking toothbrush. But nothing worked.

After 20 minutes or so, I paused to drink some water, and then I tried using my toothbrush again. It finally worked. It felt like a sweet surrender as those cookies came up. I will never forget the feeling of relief and pride I felt in that moment! I thought *Wow, I did it. And now I have the best secret because no one will have to know anything about it.*

And I was right. That fucking secret took me down to my knees!

That was the beginning of an addiction that I lived with for decades after that. When I went to college, I couldn't hide it anymore, but I did discover that alcohol could help.

Chapter 2

There's Power in Powerlessness

When I think about the first time I got drunk, all I can tell you is that it's very fuzzy. Although I don't remember much of that time of my life, I want to share bits and pieces of my story with you to show you how cunning, baffling and powerful alcohol truly is.

My relationship with alcohol really began before college, on the evening of my prom. I was living in New Jersey and had risen the social ladder. I was thin. I had friends. I was a cheerleader. In many ways, I felt like I had finally arrived. On the night of the prom, I dressed in a beautiful dress with my hair pulled back in a big, long ponytail secured with a banana clip (remember those from the 80s?) My date, Keith, and I were going to the prom in a limo with the "cool kids,". They picked me up at my house. Before we left, there were the obligatory pictures, and we stole sips of alcohol as our parents lined us up for the photos. What I remember as I think back on it now are glimpses of happiness.

But as soon as I got in the limo, I remember absolutely nothing. All I know is that the next morning I woke up in my bedroom which was full of puke, vomit and piss, and I was filled with the overwhelming feelings of shame, anger, remorse, and resentment. Someone had dropped me off at my house, put me in bed with my prom dress on, and then I woke up in that filth. To say that I was disgusted with myself was an understatement, but like a good alcoholic, that didn't stop me. Instead, I thought to myself, "Wow, did I have fun last night!" In a crazy, misguided way, it felt like a badge of honor to black out and not remember anything.

So, that was how I spent most of my senior year. Alcohol was currency. It meant I could have friends, meet boys and be popular. Just like when I was in junior high, I was always trying to fit in, and alcohol gave me a ticket to the "cool club."

When I was looking for colleges, all I knew was I wanted to get the fuck out of New Jersey, and I wanted to get the fuck away from my parents, as many kids headed to college do. That's why I picked the University of Massachusetts. It's often referred to as "The Zoo" because it is one of the biggest party schools out there. And it is so big, that it gave me the ability to hide and be anonymous. At the same time I was heading to college, my parents moved from New Jersey to Switzerland. So, on the day I had to move in, I drove all by myself to Massachusetts in my Buick Skylark. No parents. No brother or sister. I went all by myself – completely alone.

Pulling up to the dorm, I could see all the other parents helping their kids set up their rooms. And there I was, by myself. It was exactly like I had always felt—alone. So, it's no surprise that my freshman year was a complete shit show.

When I drank, I didn't have to think about my food addiction. Of course, it caused a lot of other problems, and I put myself in some really bad situations. I also lost a lot of friends.

My housemates would say, "Where's the food? Oh, Yvette ate it and threw it up."

Other people around me started to notice and ask, "Where's the food going? Where's the money? Where's the house money?"

It was embarrassing and I was filled with shame. So, I decided to leave college for a semester. I got a job and told myself I was going to get my life together. But the opposite happened. My life got into more disarray. I started drinking and throwing up all the time. Every day, I woke up and went to work as a fitness instructor at a health club. When I got done, I went to the store, and bought pancake mix. Then I made 30-40 pancakes, slathered them in butter and syrup, and ate them all. I made sure nobody was home before I threw up.

My other option would be to go to a diner or the pancake house and throw up afterward. Then I would get ready to go out and binge drink.

But it was the food that really took me down. I can't even explain the shame I felt for starving myself, then going to exercise, then eating and throwing up. I was filled with so much regret, but I kept repeating that same pattern over and over again. At the peak of my addiction, I was throwing up 8 to 10 times a day. It was awful, and the consequences started to show. I lost my hair. My teeth were rotting. I had bruises all over my body. I added extensions to cover the hair loss. I tanned to cover my bruises. I always found some way to get out of looking sick because vanity was always my number one concern. But the truth was, underneath everything, I was a freaking mess. And I looked like a freaking mess.

I did absolutely nothing academically. I didn't go to class, and I kept changing my major. First, I thought that I would be an exercise science major because I loved to exercise. But that program required chemistry, and I wasn't going to take that course. Then I thought I would try nutrition. But that required math classes which I also wasn't going to do. That's when I found Hotel, Restaurant and Travel administration. Since I figured I can bullshit like the best of them, I thought this one might be it. But in the first class, they said you had to be willing to work 100 hour weeks. Nope, that wasn't happening. Because I've always been good at finding the loopholes and manipulating the situation to find the easy way out, I eventually did earn my degree in Sports Management. But guess what? That was because it was the major that had all the cute boys. In fact, I happened to be dating one of them! He was a good-looking football player, and he was also a bouncer at a local bar. When I walked in that bar, I thought, *Man, I have arrived.*

One night, the Red Sox were playing the Mets in the World Series, and everyone was having parties on campus. The guy I was dating took me to one of the fraternity parties. I walked in thinking I was hot shit, but that didn't last long. The drinking was out of control and at some point, we ended up in a bedroom. Without getting into too many details, all I can say is that I was sexually assaulted. I tried to fight him off, and I screamed and cried for help. But nobody came. All those men in that frat house, and not one person came to help me! Eventually I fought myself free, put my underwear on and grabbed a big shirt that was on the floor. Then I ran out to the street. Thankfully, someone drove by, and they took me back to my dorm.

I never spoke about what happened. Even when I went to the university health service center to speak with a counselor, I never spoke about it. My drinking was already bad, but after that night, I started a deep, spiral descent into drinking. I had so much anger towards this guy who was supposedly my boyfriend, and I was also furious that nobody came to help me. I knew I went to his bedroom voluntarily and because of that, I had put myself into the situation. So, I figured if I told anyone, they wouldn't believe me. To this day, I'm still filled with regret, shame and remorse about it. And of course, the only way I knew how to cope was to drink and throw up.

That's when I decided to take time off from school. It's when I ended up working at the health club teaching fitness classes. Every day I was throwing up, and every night I was drinking. It's crazy to look back at it now and realize that was the life I led my whole college career.

As I said, the effects of all of the abuse were starting to show. My hair was dry, my nails were brittle, and my teeth started to turn brown. I didn't look good. So, just like I always did, I covered it up. I made myself look like Gucci on the outside, but I felt like Walmart on the inside.

I never felt a part of any of it, though. When I was in college, my parents weren't living in this country, and for every Christmas and every Thanksgiving, I had to "couch surf" to different places, always looking for someone to take me in. I lived like an orphan, and it was so hard. I tried to cover up everything that was happening. No matter where I was, I was always the one on the outside feeling like I didn't fit in. It was just such a sad and lonely existence. It felt like I had an emptiness in my soul.

The good news out of all of it is that I ended up graduating from college. My parents moved back to New Jersey, and I moved back home after college. When I was looking for a job, that's where my best thinking came to me.

Chapter 3

The Cycle

I had two interviews. One was with the M&M Company. Yep, if I got that job, I would have been a bulimic driving around with a company car filled with chocolate. Can you imagine? The second interview was to become a sales rep for a wine company—Bartles & Jaymes. I was a full-blown alcoholic bulimic looking for jobs where I could just feed my addiction daily. Needless to say, I didn't get those jobs, but that's where my head was at—just to give you an idea of how fucked up I was.

In any event, by the time I was 21, I had my own apartment, and I was selling ads for the Yellow Pages. When I visited clients, I scouted out all the diners along the way. I also looked for Dunkin' Donuts, McDonalds or any restaurants that had buffets. I knew where every private bathroom was along the route, so I could go in and throw up without anyone knowing. That was my drug for many, many years.

I was very successful. I had a company car. I won trips to Rome and Hawaii, and I was killing it in the game. But because of my drinking, I ended up losing my job. I was great at selling, but my follow through was not that great. Inevitably, my work started to deteriorate, and they told me they didn't need me anymore. On the day they fired me, my sales manager had to drive me home because I had to turn in the only car I had—the company car.

At that point I was without a job… and without a car! So, the consequences of my choices were definitely building up. But I did have some things that kept me going. I was living with a guy named Jim. He was a former customer of mine from the Yellow Pages, and he was a fireman. He was a great guy, but at this point I was drinking a lot, and he was my savior. I was living in Linden, New Jersey, and one day I went to this gym called Guys 'n Dolls. While I was there, a guy named Ivan told me not to worry. He asked me, "Why don't you just do something for fast cash for now? You'll get a job in the future someplace where you can use your languages and your college degree."

"Okay, Ivan," I said. "That sounds like a great fucking idea. What have you got?"

He says, "Why don't you go to this Go-Go bar and become a shot girl?"

"What's a shot girl?" I asked.

I don't remember what he answered, but whatever he said got me to go. I went to this Go-Go bar called Breathless, in Rahway, New Jersey. I showed up in a navy blue business suit with a pair of little kitten heels. I had no idea what the fuck I was walking into, but as soon as I arrived, I was like, "Yeah! This is my jam! Sign me up!" The lure of that club, the loud music, the people partying—it felt like just where I wanted to be. And I ended up staying in that industry for five years.

My job was basically to get up and drink with customers, and I loved it. I worked the best nights. I had the best customers. My greatest customer owned Polly-O Cheese. Whenever he came, he never tipped anybody else but me, and I never walked out with less than $1,000 to $2,000 a night. I was living the high life. Honestly, I was just a companion, a friend to this guy. He just took to me and liked my personality, and he was really a big reason I was able to sustain as long as I did. But in any event, partying and cocaine, which I'll get into later, really started to take over my life. At this point, I had tried to stop drinking and had been to maybe three or four rehabs, but every time I went to rehab, I would say, "You know what? I just need to stop doing cocaine. I'll be fine. I'll manage my drinking. I'll only drink at night. I'll only drink on the weekends, and I'll only drink wine instead of vodka."

I had every bullshit fucking negotiation with myself you can think of. This time after rehab I went back to the

Go-Go bar, and that cycle continued for countless rehabs. Eventually, I was fired from the Go-Go bar because I had a habit of not showing up. The night I was fired, I walked out of the bar to find that my car was gone. I called the cops to tell them it was stolen, but come to find out, it had actually been repossessed. And pretty soon I was also evicted from my apartment. That's what happens when you don't pay your bills!

I lived in my car for a while and got a job bartending and doing some personal training. I took showers at the gym, and then I went to work. I couch-surfed sometimes or went from motel to motel. I was so lost. Eventually I moved back home, but I was still partying a lot.

One night I was out in New York City at a club called Webster Hall, and the next morning I went to the gym to train my client, Barbara. I got there at 5:00 AM with my gym bag over my shoulder. Inside the bag, the vodka bottles clanked together so you could hear me coming from a mile away. Barbara was a beautiful, blonde woman who worked in real estate. And here I was as high as a kite, still drunk on the vodka that had been in those bottles! I told her to start giving me some pushups. I got down on the floor to do them with her, and she stopped. "Yvette," she said, "I really want to take you to my house and have a conversation with you."

So, that's what we did. I went to her house, and she sat me down and said, "I think you have a drinking problem."

I said, "What are you talking about?"

She looked at me and replied in a kind voice, "You're high right now. You're drunk. Let me take you to a recovery meeting."

And that was how I got to my first recovery meeting. I will always be grateful to Barbara because she was the first person who took the time out to say, "I want to help you, and I have no ulterior motive." Needless to say, I did not get sober that first time, but she was instrumental in my journey to sobriety.

The problem was that even when I tried to stop, I always went back to dancing and bartending. It gave me a way to make good money, and it was easy access to drugs and alcohol. It just had me hooked. Still, after a while, I ended up going to rehab again and this time when I came out, I decided that I really wanted to try and stay sober now. So, I asked my dad to put a down payment on an apartment for me. And he did. I didn't have any money for furniture, but I had a place to live in Southbound Brook. And I had a car! One of my old boyfriends had given me a car from his limo business. It was a Crown Vic – like a fucking cop car! Imagine that! Usually, I was running from the cops, but here I was driving around looking like one of them.

Chapter 4

Rock Bottom is a Solid Foundation

When I took the job as a Go Go dancer, I had to give myself a new name, so I chose "Gabriela D." The "D" stood for "Delicious." Can you imagine? When I made up the name, they wanted me to use my initial for a last name. At the time, my maiden name was Dicenta, and so my initial was "D." I had to come up with something that the "D" stood for, and I couldn't think of anything else, so I chose "D" for "Delicious." It had that catchy tone to it, I thought.

One night I was working at the bar, Cheeks. What a name! It says it all, right? Anyway, I was working, and I had definitely tipped back a few too many drinks. I was on stage with my 6" stiletto heels, wobbling around, and not looking very attractive. When I got done with my set, the bartender pulled me over and said, "I think you need a bump."

I wasn't sure what she meant. A bump, like a fist bump? I had no idea about anything to do with the drug world. I was completely naive to the whole thing.

She said, "I'll meet you in the bathroom."

When we got there, she rolled up a dollar bill, went over to the aluminum toilet paper holder and laid out a line of coke. She crushed it up with a credit card, and then handed me the dollar bill. She said, "Just sniff this."

I said, "All right, let's do it."

Almost immediately, I had the most incredible feeling. I can't explain it completely, but it was as if I'd been living in a bland world, and all of a sudden, somebody put the lights on — every light, every color, just brightly shining and flashing and explosive fireworks as it all flooded through my brain.

That was my first experience with cocaine, but it wasn't the last. I chased that high for a long, long time.

On that night, though, I went back on stage, and I pulled off power moves I never thought were possible. I did tricks on the pole that I never thought I had the strength to do. The cocaine gave me some kind of superpower. The owner of a local business, John, was there that night, and he gave me a standing ovation. A "Standing O" in the Go-Go World is called "Let it Rain" meaning they stop the music and pour dollar bills over the dancer — $100s, $50s or $5s.

So, there I was, on the floor doing my dance move on my knees, and "swimming" around in the dollar bills. I was picking up fifties and hundreds on the freaking dance stage, and all I could think was, *Let's go. This is a good time! It's a total score!* And another part of my brain was thinking, I need to marry the cartel dealer right now! I never want to go a day without this shit!

I left the bar that night, and when I got home, I thought, *How am I going to get more of this?* And that became the chase. I wanted every night to be like that one, and I ended up spending the next five years chasing it.

I found people who had blow and who partied like I did, and after work, I went out with them. My life started to spiral really quickly. In one way, I am grateful that I was a cocaine user because it is the kind of drug that brings you to your knees so much faster than alcohol. I could have been a functioning alcoholic for another 20 years, but the cocaine did me in much more quickly. I was losing shit left and right, and I was spending a crazy amount of money — between $250 to $400 a day on cocaine.

When people say, "I can't hire an addict," I tell them, "Are you fucking kidding me? Addicts will wake up with absolutely no business plan and figure out a way to make $300 or $400 in just a few hours!"

And that's what I did on the daily. Of course, it also started to have an effect on my dancing. I went from working nights to working days. Thursday, Friday, and Saturday nights were the time to earn the most money because it's when there were bachelor parties. That's when the "big players" showed up. But I went from working nights to working Mondays at noon, and let me tell you, the characters who come to a Go-Go bar during the daytime are fucking sad.

But that's where the drug took me. I had no money to eat, and I would wait for 4:00 when they would serve nasty hot dogs at the bar. Can you imagine sitting at the bar with some creeper, in my high heels and shorts, eating some nasty 20-day-old hot dogs? Yeah, not so pretty. But that was my life. And still I kept chasing it!

There are many, many crazy stories. One of them is when I went to audition for another Go-Go bar in Staten Island called Lipsticks. My job in New Jersey wasn't going well. I could tell they were starting to be unhappy with my work and thought I might get fired. I figured I might as well try to get a job at another place. So, I drove out to Staten Island and got there about 10:00 PM. On the way, I saw a guy hitchhiking. Now mind you, I'm a woman by myself at that hour, and still, I stopped the car and let the guy get in. He said, "Where are you going?"

I said, "I'm going to Lipsticks."

He smiled and said, "Well, in that case, I've got a proposition for you. How about me and you just party as buddies, and let's just fucking have a good time? Whatever you would've made at Lipsticks, I'll pay you."

I thought about it for a split second, and told him, "Sure. I'll do it for $500" which is what I figured I would have made that night anyway.

He agreed and took me to a motel. We were partying our faces off. In fact, I think I might've smoked crack, but I was so fucked up, I didn't even know that's what it was. All I know is I smoked it out of a Budweiser bottle. I put a rock on top and he said, "Just blow here." I absolutely had no idea what I was doing.

A couple of hours later, there was a knock on the door. When I opened it, there was a huge 6'2" man standing there with a rifle underneath his trench coat. My mind scrambled to figure out what the fuck was going on here. The guy behind me and the guy at the door seemed to have some kind of beef with each other, and I thought, *This is my exit.* I grabbed my things and told him to give me my $500. I wasn't leaving until I got the money that he had promised me. I was like a 5-year-old who had been promised gum on the playground! *You promised to give it to me!*

Still, miraculously, he gave me the money, and I got out of there as fast as I could. I drove back to Linden, New Jersey thinking, *Man, this is getting a little scary.*

But my head was so messed up that by the time I got home, I was already telling myself, *It's not that bad. You've got Cheeks. You've got Uncle Charlie's, and you've got Bourbon Street. Just stay away from Staten Island.*

That's what my life was like. I was always justifying and negotiating, trying to find a different way to manage my drinking and my drugging. If somebody asked me, "Are you holding?" My answer would always be, "Yeah, I'm holding, but I'm not sharing, motherfucker. The shit is for me."

In the drug world, it became all about "what are you going to do for me? And if you're not doing something for me, I'm not doing anything for you."

I used to play tricks on myself. I would tell myself I wasn't going to use it all at one time. I promised myself I was going to save some for later when I got home from work. Then I hid the baggies to keep it away from me.

One night, I hid the baggie in the base of a plant holder. When I got home from work, I couldn't remember where it was, and I tore my apartment apart. I even sniffed the carpet looking for pebbles of coke. Yeah, now that's attractive!

Even though I knew it was out of control, and I told myself I had to stop, I didn't.

I had a really great high school friend named Camber. We met at a bar, and she actually came to see me at the Go-Go bar. She said, "Good Lord! What the fuck happened to you, Yvette?"

And I said, "Oh no, sister. It's Gabriela D from here on in. Look how popular I am. Look how much money I have."

Meanwhile, this girl had her shit together. We had been through a lot together, but that night, she left the bar. She was disappointed in me and that really hurt. She told me I could do better, and she was right. But I couldn't see that then. I was still lost in the life I had created for myself.

At one point I met a golden gloves boxer named Henry. We hit it off, and I actually ended up living with him for a while. Here are how our two brains worked. We woke up each day and did a workout that consisted of skipping rope and then running. When we got home, we did three or four lines, then we'd hit the heavy bag at the gym together. And we'd finish the day by drinking all night. He was a professional boxer, and our "best" training consisted of running, skipping, doing blow, going back to the gym and hitting the heavy bag, and then drinking all night and watching movies. He really, really loved me, but I am sorry to say that the story didn't end so well with him. Recently, I looked him up to see if he was still alive, and I learned he had actually been stabbed to death. That's where this disease takes you.

But in any event, I ended up leaving Henry, and ultimately, I realized that I had to get clean. Still, it took a while. One day I was at a tavern, and it got out of hand. I did too much, but once you've done it, you can't take it back. My heart started racing, and I felt like I was going to have a heart attack. It was too much, and I wanted it to stop, but there wasn't anything I could do. I tried to steady my breathing, I went to the bathroom and tried to walk it off. Thankfully, my heart rate eventually slowed down, and I could breathe normally again.

One morning a few months later, I went to the bathroom and did a line. Suddenly, my nose started bleeding. I stuck my pinky fingers up my nose to see what was in there. One was in each nostril, and I could actually touch my fingers together. I had blown a hole right through my nose. And that's when I finally hit rock bottom! I am as vain as fuck, and I was not going to have a collapsed nose, like Michael Jackson, because of my drug use. I was 30 years old, and I was done with cocaine. My vanity stopped me!

The good news is that I stopped. The bad news is that I lost five years of my life. It wasn't a complete blackout because I do have bits and pieces of memories. But it was definitely a brownout, and I'm sorry I don't remember more.

I don't think many people can do cocaine recreationally. I think a lot of people like to sell themselves a bill of goods that they're just going to do it once in a while. But it really is the gateway drug to so many things. First of all, doing cocaine means you won't think about food. Secondly, it makes you feel beautiful, attractive, outgoing, and like the life of the party. And the third thing is that it has no calories. Because of all those reasons, it had me hooked.

I just want you to know that if you're struggling with cocaine or any other drug, my best advice is to recognize what's going on. Step outside of your day-to-day and ask yourself, "Is this the life I really want to live?" If the answer is no, then get help.

Let's talk about the real cost of blow. It's like lighting your wallet on fire and dancing around the bonfire, except the fire is your life going up in smoke. We're not just talking about blowing your dough on powder; the real bankruptcy is in the currency of relationships, mental health, and everything that makes life worth living.

And here's the real kicker — that first high? It's the best you'll ever feel. From that point on, you're chasing! All day, every day you're trying to get back to the way it felt the first time. What's worse is that every hit takes you further from the prize, not closer. You end up in a loop of shame and regret where the stakes are your sanity, your health, and maybe your life. And it's all for the thrill of the chase that's as empty as the baggie at the end of the night.

I know if I pick up a drink or a drug, I will lose myself again, and I don't want that. I want to be here for my kids. It's the most important aspect of my life. And I will never put cocaine up my nose because I believe my nose will collapse. It's the story I've told myself since I was 30, and I'm sticking to it because it's kept me clean from cocaine.

Although I surrendered to cocaine for a few years of my life, I am so grateful that it brought me to the bottom so fast. Because rock bottom is a solid foundation!

Chapter 5

Sick and Tired of Being Sick and Tired

In my late 20's, I was really struggling, however I also wanted to get better. I wanted to stop throwing up and I was trying to get sober. So, in order to stay sober, I applied for a job at the Home News Tribune to sell advertising. One day while I was out selling ads, I walked into a bagel store and asked to see the owner. Apparently, he wasn't there, so I could have come back later. But standing there looking at that food was making me hungry. And I didn't have any money for food. Something in my brain clicked, and I thought, "I'm just going to steal a muffin." And I did. That's how bad things had become. I didn't have any furniture or money for food, but I always managed to find a way.

Soon after that, though, the guy who owned the bagel shop asked me out. His name was Dave. My first thought was, "Why not? At least I'll get a free meal." So, we went out to eat and had a fun night. There is much more to share about Dave, but you'll have to wait to read it in the next chapter.

But after that night out with him, I went to work the next day. When I walked in, my manager, Brenda, asked me to come into her office. I was doing well in my job and was the #1 sales rep, so I thought I was going in there to be promoted. Instead, she sat me down and said, "We think you have a drinking problem, and we want you to go into an Employee Assistance Program."

In my mind, I'm thinking, *Brenda, what the fuck are you telling me? You've got some kind of balls to talk to me like that.* But at the same time, I was holding a Dunkin' Donuts coffee cup filled with vodka. That's where my thinking was at that point! It was messed up!

I took her advice, though, and entered an intensive out-patient rehab program. It was really the only option, but the interesting thing is that this was the first rehab I had been in where I actually started to listen. It's the first time I thought that maybe alcohol was one of my problems.

At that time, I was still throwing up and drinking a lot. And I said, "You know what? I'm tired of this. I'm sick and tired of trying to manage my drinking and feeling like shit all the time. And then finding myself drunk every morning with the remorse, shame, and guilt." I was just tired. So, I did that intensive outpatient voluntarily, and I actually listened and went to recovery meetings.

There was a meeting in New Brunswick that I went to where I didn't know anyone. I was scared, but I forced myself to go in. They asked if there was anyone new at the meeting that night, and I raised my hand. "I'm new," I said, "and I need help."

A woman named Patti answered, "I'll help you."

And that is when I met the angel who saved my life!

Patti Maloney is her name, and I will always be grateful to her. Before meeting Patti I had never met anyone who did things with no ulterior motive. It truly blew my mind away. She was that kind of person who would pick me up and take me to meetings, answer my calls, and take me out for coffee to show me this new way of life.

In recovery they say…"Find somebody who has what you want." I definitely wanted what she had.

In 12-step recovery, our sole purpose is to help another, but I did not realize that at the time. I never understood it. *Like really? That's how you stay sober??!*

But that's the truth. That's how you stay sober—by helping another person who is still sick and suffering. Crazy, right? But that's how it works!

Patti looks like an angel, but let me tell you, she is definitely hard-core. I remember at the beginning of my sobriety I called her up wasted out of my mind and said, "Patti, I love you so much. Let's let this whole recovery thing go, and let's go out together. We will have such a blast."

She quickly told me to call her when I was sober and that she didn't have time for any of that.

Ouch!!!!!!!

I truly think that memory sticks out so clearly in my mind because she meant so much to me. No one had ever believed in me like she did. She just kept telling me, over and over, "If you keep doing the next right thing, buckle up…you will have a life beyond your wildest dreams!"

And I don't know why, but I did believe her!

Patti is an amazing woman! She has a beautiful gift. She's an amazing musician. I never understood how she could perform in bars around alcohol, but she explained to me that if you go through this program and live it one day at a time, you can go anywhere as long as you are spiritually fit. And like I said, for some reason, I believed her.

Trying to get sober was hard because I had spent so much time on drinking and drugging that I literally didn't even know what to do with myself. I remember being home on a Friday night, bored out of my mind, and she told me to scrub my floors in the kitchen, go to a meeting or go to the gym. She was instrumental in my recovery, truly. I did not know how to live. I did not know how to show up. I did not know how to care for others.

Patti literally lives the program, and it's because of her that I am alive today.

Getting sober is hard! If it was not for this 12-step program, I definitely would not have stayed sober. It's amazing to think that June 29, 2003…. I got sober and have maintained that sobriety!

It wasn't my first go around, but I'll explain more about that later. Still, joining a 12-step program gave me new friends, a purpose, community, and a design for living. It may not be for everyone but, for sure, it changed my entire life.

Chapter 6

Life's a Bitch, and Then You Meet a Man Named Dave

Let me pause for a moment to tell you more about my husband, Dave. Yep, the owner of the bagel store. He was definitely put on my path to save my life. As I was slowly trying to kill myself, God had a different plan. He decided to put a man in my life who believed in me, and because I've experienced this, I am so adamant about having someone in your life who believes in you. You need support, and you need that one person who's going to say, no matter what, "We're going to get through this!"

So how did I meet Dave? At this point I had one foot in the Go-Go world working at night, and one foot in the corporate world trying to sell advertising for a paper called The Home News Tribune. As I mentioned in the last chapter, I was at a point where I was trying to stay sober with an emphasis on the word "trying." I wasn't fully committed because

I was caught between the world of fast cash and also trying to do the "right thing."

So, when I walked into a bagel store to see if they wanted to buy advertising for the paper and the owner wasn't there, I stole a muffin when the guy at the counter turned away. It smelled so good, and I was so hungry that I just took it. It's crazy to think that I stole a muffin from a man who later became my husband! But more on that in a minute.

Since the owner wasn't there, I left with my muffin and proceeded to go to the liquor store. At that time, I was drinking 3-4 airplane-size bottles of vodka in the morning. Needless to say, by 11:00 a.m., I was done with work!

A couple of days later, I got a call at the paper from a man named Dave. He said he was the owner of the bagel store. At first I thought he was going to say something about the muffin, but instead he said, "I hear that you're kind of cute, and I'd like to take you out to dinner."

My first response was, "I don't want to go out to dinner. I really just want you to buy an ad for the paper!"

Without hesitating, he said, "I'll sign up for an ad if you go out to dinner with me."

That sounded like a good deal to me—I made a sale and was going to get some free food, too! Perfect! So, we went out to dinner in Somerset, New Jersey at a restaurant called La Primavera. We decided to meet at the restaurant and when I saw him, I was in shock. His clean-cut, American, apple pie image was not my usual go-to. He showed up clean shaven and wore rimmed glasses! This man looked very smart. Definitely not my go-to con man! Immediately I thought, *Oh no, I don't know about this*. But we ended up having dinner and had such a great conversation that we were the last ones to leave the restaurant. They were sweeping the floor around us as we left. Of course, the thing was, we had a great time because 1) he was paying; and 2) we drank multiple bottles of wine.

Afterward, he came back to my apartment to hang out. When he walked in the door, he hesitated as he looked around the empty room. "Where's your furniture?" he asked.

I laughed it off and said, "Oh, the furniture is getting delivered." It wasn't true, of course. In reality, I didn't have any furniture, and my bed was just a mattress on the floor. Fortunately, he didn't seem to be that bothered about the furniture. He was more affected by the heat. In fact, he said the apartment was so hot that he ended up buying an air conditioner for me.

A couple days after our date, he sent me six dozen roses at work. Although I was impressed and thought he was a great guy, my mind was definitely not clear at that time. Rather than realizing that I had found a gem, I was thinking that I needed to get this sucker over to the Go-Go bar so I could loosen him and rape him for his money.

Thankfully, that's not what happened. Instead, that was when my manager pulled me into the office to tell me that I needed to go to the Employee Assistance Program because she thought I had a drinking problem. Sitting there with a Dunkin' Donuts cup filled with vodka, I had the balls to argue with her that she was wrong, but she didn't give up. She gave me an ultimatum—either get help or you're fired.

So, I got help, and that was the one rehab that actually stuck. Looking back on it now, I think I stuck to it not just because I was tired of the merry-go-round rehab circuit, but also because of Dave. All my other friends and my family had deserted me, but he stuck with me. He was a lifeline to hold onto.

After I was released into the outpatient program, I went to my first 12-step program recovery meeting. After the meeting, I told Dave that I really needed to stop drinking. Then I gave him an ultimatum. I told him that if he wanted to be a part of my life, he had to stop, too. Talk about balls! Here I am telling this grown man that he's got to stop drinking so that he can stay with me. And his prize will be a 30-year-old woman with absolutely no financial means, no furniture, no car, and no job. He had every reason to walk away, but he didn't. Instead, he got sober, too. He told me,

"I believe in you, so let's do it together." And to this day, he's never picked up a drink again. As you're going to read in the next chapter, that was not the case for me, but still, together we made progress.

After 30 days, I got my sober coin, and after the meeting, he was waiting for me. As I got in the car, he handed me a little brown bag. I could smell the delicious bagel inside, and I loved his bagels so I couldn't wait to open it. Inside the bag was a shellacked bagel with the words "Will you marry me?" on it. I'll never forget that car ride! I couldn't believe it. All I could think was, *Are you for real? You really want to marry me?*

And he did, and so we did. In rehab they tell you that you shouldn't make any major changes within the first year of sobriety, but I'm not one to follow rules. So, within the first four months of being sober, I was engaged to be married to a stranger who believed that I was his prize. He was an amazing man. Within a few months, we bought our first condo, and he put my name on the deed. I didn't even own a car, but thanks to him, now I owned a condo. He also let me drive his sports car, getting a beat-up car for himself. In other words, he always put me first.

I am forever grateful to this man who played a huge role in saving my life. What I realize is that no one can get you out of addiction alone. You need to be surrounded with people who believe in you. These people always believed in me.

I would never have gotten sober without God, Patti, my recovery community, and Dave.

Chapter 7

Relapse… Back to Basics

So, at this point in my journey, I'm three years sober. It's 2003, and life is going okay. I am free from alcohol and drugs, and I'm teaching my fitness class. I am married with a baby on the way. Life is going great.

But then, here it comes…drumroll, please…the relapse.

It's really important for me to write about relapse because I feel like there is so much shame and stigma around it! There are actually statistics out there that 80% of the people who end up getting sober through a 12-step program will not go back if they relapse! I'm grateful that wasn't me.

They always say a relapse happens before it happens. The disease is literally doing push-ups, getting stronger, and waiting for a weak moment. And that's exactly what happened to me.

I had all the material things back, and I became a little too busy. I got too busy to go to meetings or to call my sponsor. I didn't have any urges to drink, I just thought life was happening and everything was good…until it wasn't.

It was June 29, 2003. My niece was having a graduation party in her backyard, and I figured the least I could do was get a bottle of wine for the host. Right there…that's the red flag. I had not entered a liquor store in three years.

Really, Yvette? Couldn't you get her a plant?

But no…the stinkin' thinkin' got the best of me.

So, I went to the liquor store, got the bottle of wine for the host, and went to the party.

It was a beautiful day outside, but all I could remember focus on were these Solo cups everyone was holding. I don't know why that triggered me, but I just had the great idea that if I got a Solo cup, nobody would know if I put wine or Kool-Aid in it. So, I did exactly that. I filled up a Solo cup with wine, and I had my first chug. And it felt glorious… fuckin' glorious! Never mind that at this time I was seven months pregnant. This is where my best thinking got me.

I had the time of my life at that party, but honestly as the party went on, I don't remember much. What I do remember is that my daughter's name was supposed to be Emily, and instead, it is now Mary Rose. So, there's that.

How did that happen? Well, it happened because in my drunken stupor. I was joking around with my mother-in-law whose name is Mary, and I decided to say how amazing she was and how my daughter would be honored to have her name, blah blah blah, and then I stuck a rose at the end of it because why not have it be like a flower? And that's how I named my daughter, Mary Rose.

Crazy! Just like that. I do think to this day that her name is the reminder I need about what was really happening in that moment. I love the name Mary Rose, and I'm so grateful that my daughter's name is Mary Rose, but really?!! Rest in peace, Emily.

So I continued to drink and then went home to bed. I never wanted to talk about it again. My husband did not know, but I knew, and I carried extreme shame. I mean you're seven months pregnant, Yvette. Really? You're going to drink alcohol now while you have a baby in your body? What the fuck is wrong with you?

"What the fuck wrong" is addiction? Addiction is a disease that tells, "you don't have a disease." It's a disease that's waiting for that one weak moment so it can climb in and fuck up your whole life. But because I had been going to recovery meetings for three years, I knew it was best to tell my sponsor.

The first rule of thumb…secrets keep you sick!

Second rule…always keep your side of the street clean.

So, I did exactly that. I called Patti and said, "Listen. I'm so ashamed, but I drank last night. It was only for one day. I don't think I need to tell Dave or anyone else for that matter."

That was a big fat no!

She explained to me that in order to stay sober, you have to be vigorously honest with yourself and with others. "You are going to have to go back to the meetings and raise your hand and say you're coming back, and you have to tell your husband," she said. Double gulp!!

"But Patti, it was only a slip. It wasn't even a full day. And Dave doesn't even know."

"That's not the point. If you don't want to continue to drink, and you want to get sober again, you have to start from day one. This is just a learning lesson. You took your foot off the pedal. You started to coast. And this is what happens. How can you grow from this?"

I hated questions like that. How can I grow from this? I don't wanna go back and raise my hand. There's so much shame in that. But I did exactly that! I told my husband that I drank, and I went back to the recovery meetings and raised my hand.

And here's the thing, after that meeting, so many people came up to me and said I might've saved them from relapsing. So, by sharing my experience maybe I was able to help somebody else who was considering having "just one." That's how recovery works. It's not just about me. It's about helping others! When I am honest, and I help others, that's what keeps me sober. That's what the whole program is based on. Had I not been going to this program, I probably would've kept drinking.

This relapse showed me so much. It gave me a lesson in humility. Recovery literally is "one day at a time." The gift that recovery has given me is the understanding and acceptance that this is a battle I will have for the rest of my life. You're never cured. You never graduate!

The other lesson it showed me is gratitude. I am so grateful to not have to pick up and use every day to handle my emotions. I understand that detours happen in life, and all you can do is learn from it. Learning to be compassionate with myself and having gratitude to be able to come back is huge!!! Many people that relapse never make it back. I know what's waiting for me if I go back out...jail, institutions, and death. Thank you, God, for giving me the gift to sobriety.

Chapter 8

Releasing my Last Demon… Food

I've written a lot about what it was like with drugs and alcohol, but I want to circle back to the food because this one is super sneaky. First of all, food is legal! So, there's that. Plus, we also need food to survive. We just can't quit food. We have to manage food.

For somebody who is an addict, who is all in or all out, it's very hard to manage anything. I also think that many people don't talk about their food struggles because it's like, "Really? You got taken down by a brownie?!"

But yes, motherfucker as a matter, fact, I did. It's just that my "brownie" was pancakes!!

So at this point in my life, I had given up the drinking and drugging. It was 2016, and I was 47 years old, and I was bulimic. I was definitely not bulimic like I was in my younger years, but I couldn't go 90 days without throwing up. That was my goal every time I threw up. I restarted my day count. But I could never get 90 days.

I did get a reprieve, though, because I had used all the tools from my 12-step program towards food addiction. But it was still present in my life, and I really wanted to be done with it! I was tired of being sick and tired. I had been on this hamster wheel since I was 14.

I would get sick and tired and tell myself, *That's it. I'm never doing this again.* And then I would forget how bad it was and get right back on the cycle. The worst for me was dealing with the shame of imposter syndrome. At this point in my life, I was really into heavy weight training, and I was this image of fitness. But I really wasn't. Nobody knew the secret. I would go on photo shoots with my eight-pack, and nobody would know the turmoil in my brain. It's the one thing that I always say about mental health. It's not visible to the eye. Nobody would have ever thought that I was sticking my head in a toilet bowl where people shit. Yet I was, and I was doing it at the same time I was being photographed for a magazine cover.

As I write this, I think, *Wow, that was bonkers!*

The other shameful part about being bulimic is that it's dirty. At least with anorexia, it's all built up on willpower. I'm anorexic. I have willpower. But bulimia, it's like you don't have willpower and you're disgusting. At least, those were the beliefs that were in my head.

Food was my best friend since I was 14 years old. It was my comfort and my entertainment. It always did what it was supposed to do. It never failed me. Bulimia gave me that instant gratification. That relief of being able to get rid of it all. What a vicious cycle!

We all have those moments...those defining moments where we need to make a change. For me, that came on an average Wednesday afternoon when I was home alone.

I was done with work, and I was home. I was alone which is when all my binging and purging happened. I had binged on 30 pancakes or even more, and I felt so sick. I went to the bathroom to throw up, but nothing was coming up. The balloon bag at the back of my throat was raw and red from gagging and gagging, but still, nothing would come up. I felt completely helpless on that cold bathroom floor.

But like all good addicts, I didn't give up. After a few more tries, I was able to throw up, but one thing happened. I could not swallow. I literally could not swallow. I was scared for the very first time in my life. *Am I going to die here on this bathroom floor? Should I call an ambulance? Maybe it'll go away. It's not going away. Fuck! Fuck! Fuck!!*

I don't know if it was a white light moment or God, but at that moment. I decided I needed to do something different. I knew I was going to end up dead. I just knew it. The gig was finally up.

I told my husband, and I shared with him that I was interested in attending a Tony Robbins event called Unleash the Power Within. It was something that was speaking to me and my soul that I had to go to this event. *You have to go to this!* And so, I did. It was November 2016, and I went on a plane by myself to Dallas. I was scared, afraid, and alone, but I knew I had to face my fear. Fear is an acronym in recovery for two things: Fuck Everything And Run or Face Everything And Recover. I was ready to face myself.

So at this event, Tony did a deep hypnosis. You have to imagine 10,000 people standing up and going through a deep hypnosis together. It was wild. He started to talk about if you were to continue the behaviors that you're doing now, what will happen to your life in five years? In 10 years? And 15 years? And all you could hear were 10,000 souls crying and screaming in pain. For me, my vision was seeing my two children at my gravesite saying, "Mom, it didn't have to be this way. We love you. We miss you." And that moment changed everything for me.

I came back from the event. I went to a therapist and got some medication. I attended two therapy sessions. I threw up one other time, and I can say since February 2017, I have been clean from bulimia. That is the miracle of all miracles!

I learned many lessons through the 30 years of my bulimic journey. The first lesson I would like to share with you is understanding your triggers. For me, it was stress, body image, and trauma. It wasn't until I was able to do a deep dive into those issues that I started to recover.

The second lesson for me was getting support. No matter how ashamed I was of my behavior, I always spoke to my sponsor. I'm grateful for the 12-step recovery program I had from drugs and alcohol because it taught me to truly be rigorously honest with myself and with someone else!

The third lesson for me was about changing people, places, and things. When I first started counting days without bulimia, I had to eat in front of people. I could not put myself in an environment where I could possibly slip. I also had to remove some foods. To this day I still don't eat pancakes. I'm forever scarred. I only go to places where I feel comfortable, always have my own car, and leave when it gets weird. Being addicted to food, drugs, and alcohol is pretty much all things social so I'm very aware of that.

Lesson 4 — find a replacement habit that is good for you. For me, it was weight training. I can honestly tell you that weight training saved my life! It wasn't like aerobics where I was trying to burn calories for hours on end. This was about strengthening my body. This was about showing up. This was about creating discipline and consistency in my life.

The after effect was that I got strong muscles and a toned body, but I did this completely because I needed something to do with my time. I needed something that would make me feel accomplished. Strength training did that for me!

Chapter 9

The Game Changer...
Life Coaching

During COVID, I felt really stuck. I was lonely in my marriage. I felt burnt out with my job as a fitness studio owner, and I was just feeling lost. Maybe you can relate. Have you ever just felt stuck? Maybe you feel that it's not that bad that you want to do something about it, and also good enough to make you wanna stay where you are!

It makes me think of that sentence, "It's not that bad." That sentence stuck with me for a lot of years.

How you can have all the things? A good husband? Two beautiful kids? A successful business? Your sobriety? And still feel so alone?!

Well, you can! How do I know? Because that was me!

Life coaching is something that had always spoken to me. I wanted to figure out "the answer" since I was a young girl in my 20s. I was a personal development junkie! I fig-ured, *I'm so fucked up, maybe I can find the answer in a book, a course, or a cassette.* Remember those??

Well, I had done all the research on life coaching and this one day, I just decided to press "play," put up the big dollars and show up. And that's what I did. I signed up for an online life coaching course for a full year through IPEC Life Coaching. To say I was scared was an understatement. I was afraid I was too old…I had fear I couldn't study or stay focused…I had fear that I wouldn't follow through like I had so many other times…I had fear I wouldn't have the time… Fear, fear, fear!

But honestly, I was my very first client. It taught me so much about how to think, how to feel, and how to act. It showed me all the things that we can control with our brain.

Imagine if someone would have pulled us out freshman year and said, "Take this course. It's going to teach you how to think on purpose." Imagine how much better we would all be! I honestly didn't even know it was an option to think "on purpose." I always just thought this was the way I was, and this is the way it is. What I know now is that it doesn't have to be that way at all.

Looking at your thoughts can be a very scary thing. It's almost like pulling out a couch and seeing what's been ac-cumulating under there for years and years. That's what it felt like looking into my brain. I always say it's a bad neighborhood up there. But you can't change what you don't acknowledge, and you can't acknowledge you're thinking if you don't look at it. So if you want to get better, you have to look at it.

I think a lot of us don't want to look at our thinking. Instead, we live a life on auto pilot... Head down doing the next thing... Not ever coming up for air asking, *Does this make me happy? Is this something I wanna believe anymore?*

Before I did a deep dive into life coaching, I had so many limiting beliefs. "Limiting beliefs" is just a fancy term for stories that we tell ourselves!

For so many years, the story I was telling myself was that I was unworthy fat, ugly, and disgusting. Can you imagine? Yeah, that's the thought that was running through my head for years!!!

The best life changing lesson for me through coaching was that we have the option to choose our thoughts on a daily basis. Because when we *think* differently, we *feel* differently, and we *do* differently.

When I heard that sentence, "your thinking creates your feelings," I was completely flabbergasted. Like, what??! But it's true. And you can do, it, too.

For example, I know many people who are very ashamed that they are an alcoholic or addict.

For me, I choose to think differently.

I am grateful to be a recovering alcoholic because it gives me a feeling of hope that I can help someone else. That's why I choose to recover out loud!

I used to wake up at four in the afternoon, do a line, drink my big glass of wine, get ready for work, go to work, come home in the morning, make pancakes, throw up, go to sleep, and press repeat…again and again and again. Now my life is completely different. I wake up at 4:00 AM to write in my journal. Then I work out and go to my studio to show up for my clients. In this book you've read about the crazy life I lived. But, now let me tell you about the amazing life that sobriety has given me.

I remember my sponsor, Patti, saying, "Yvette, buckle up because you're going to go on the ride of your life when you get sober. And I can't even express to you how true that is."

Now my life is filled with friends, sobriety, fitness, and a business where I get to help incredible women become stronger. I never would have dreamed it would be possible to show up for work on time and give people my undivided attention. But that was then, and this is now. Now I have 21 years of sobriety, and removing the shame and stigma around addiction is my purpose.

So, if you're struggling with addiction, with grief, with anything…you can't do it alone. You need to get vulnerable and allow other people in to help you. My two biggest take-aways from everything I've experienced in my life are:

1. We are not pre-programmed in any certain way which means that YES, you can change! You are absolutely 100% able to change your life if you are willing to.

And…

2. Your thoughts create your feelings, and your feelings create your actions. That one sentence changed my life because it's not about anything other than your thinking. Your thinking is what's going to make you choose to pick up a drink or go to a meeting. It's all about the thoughts in your head. And if you can start noticing what your thoughts are, then you can start changing them. Start reinforcing them with different behaviors, and that's when you will see that your life can change.

If you're feeling hopeless, I want you to know that if you want to change, *you can*. If you want to make your life better, *you can*. If you are ready to take a step toward a new life, *you can*. I am living proof that it is possible.

Sharing my experience, strength, and hope with you all has been an honor. I appreciate you for reading this book, and if you are suffering in silence, feel free to reach out. We can, and do, recover.

Journal Prompts

If you're struggling with addiction, please feel free to email me at yvettesalvafitness@gmail.com. If you're struggling, and I can help in any way or direct you to any resources, I will. My purpose is to help anyone that is suffering.

Another way to begin is to take some time to self-reflect and write your thoughts on paper. Here are five questions that I think are worth thinking about. I encourage you to pull out a journal and write your answers to them. If you think it…ink it. I promise it will give you so much clarity

1. **What are you struggling with right now?**

   What do you need to stop doing?

   What do you need to start doing?

2. **How has this behavior affected your daily life?**

   Relationships…

   Finances…

   Health…

3. **If you were not using drugs and alcohol, what would your daily life look like?**

4. **When using or doing that specific behavior, drinking drugging or binging, what need are you trying to fulfill?** Many times we do it because we are hungry, angry, angry, lonely, or tired!

5. **What action step could you take right now…this very minute…to turn the ship around?**

Resources

1. Alcoholics Anonymous (AA):
   - Website: https://www.aa.org/
   - Phone: You can find local AA hotlines through their website.

2. Narcotics Anonymous (NA):
   - Website: https://www.na.org/
   - Phone: NA also provides local helpline numbers on their website.

3. Overeaters Anonymous (OA):
   - Website: https://oa.org/
   - Phone: OA offers a Find a Meeting tool on their website to locate local meetings and contact info

For more information on the services Yvette offers and for additional worksheets and free resources to help you continue your journey, visit:

https://yvettesalvafitness.com/

or

https://yvettesalvacoaching.com

You can follow Yvette on:

FB or IG: @ yvettesalvafitness

Yvette is also available for speaking engagements.

Keynote:

**From Hell to Happiness:
3 Steps to Change Your Life**

To schedule a presentation, email Yvette at:

yvettesalvafitness@gmail.com

Acknowledgements

- I'd like to thank my higher power, whom I choose to call GOD. Thank you for keeping me alive and safe. Thank you for allowing me to be open to this gift of sobriety. Thank you for giving me purpose.

- Thank you to my beautiful Dave, Mary Rose, and Steven. I have been bombarding you with ideas for the last five years about writing this book. Thank you for always believing in me and for your unwavering support.

- Thank you, Todd Durkin, my mentor for five years. You always kept this book alive in me. So many times I wanted to quit, but you would remind me of the vision… and just kept dropping the title of this book at random events. You kept the dream alive for me. Thank you!

- To Kelli Watson, how it is possible that this is an actual book? Your endless patience and encouragement helped me get here. You never gave up on me and pushed me to keep talking, recording my thoughts. It's crazy to think that all those audio notes became this book. Your ability to mirror your clients' needs is truly a gift, and you have the patience and tolerance of a saint. Thank you, and I love you.

- Thank you, Chad Cannon, for guiding me, showing up, and keeping me accountable on this journey. You are a great book coach.

- Thank you, Patti Maloney, my sponsor and dearest friend. It's because of you that I found this way of life. You've been dealing with me for over 23 years—through all my crazy! Thank you for loving me and being there for me always.

- Thank you, mom and dad, for always finding me help when I was suffering. I am grateful to both of you. I am truly sorry for all I put you through.

All profits from this book will be donated to
the Todd Durkin IMPACT Foundation in memory of
Sean Rocco Vogel. Although this book is not specifically
about suicide, I understand that suicide is the final stop
for people who aren't able to find help. I am passionate
about helping people with mental health issues so they can
get the support they need before they get to that point.